# <u>Living</u> <u>with</u> <u>Chronic</u> <u>Kidney</u> <u>Disease</u> - A Journey to Wellness

Marles pearl

Living with Chronic Kidney Disease - A Journey to Wellness

Table of Contents: Living with Chronic Kidney Disease - A Journey to Wellness

# 11. Embracing the Journey to Wellness with CKD

## 11.1 Empowering Yourself for a Fulfilling Life

# Introduction

Living with Chronic Kidney Disease (CKD) can present numerous challenges, but it is also an opportunity to empower yourself and lead a fulfilling life. CKD is a chronic condition that affects the kidneys' ability to function properly, requiring ongoing management and lifestyle adjustments. However, with the right knowledge, support, and mindset, individuals with CKD can navigate these challenges and take control of their health and well-being.

In this guide, we will explore various aspects of living with CKD and provide insights, strategies, and resources to empower you along your journey. From understanding the impact of CKD on daily life to managing diet and nutrition, incorporating exercise, and addressing emotional and psychological challenges, we will cover a wide range of topics relevant to your well-being. Additionally, we will delve into treatment options, including medications, dialysis, and kidney transplantation, and discuss preventive measures and early intervention to slow down the progression of CKD.

By embracing lifestyle changes, managing symptoms, and accessing appropriate support systems, you can create a supportive environment that enhances your quality of life. We will also explore complementary therapies, such as acupuncture, yoga, and mindfulness practices, as well as the importance of creating a positive and resilient mindset. Moreover, we will provide guidance on navigating challenges related to work, travel, and maintaining a balanced lifestyle.

Throughout this guide, we aim to empower you to take an active role in your health, make informed decisions, and cultivate resilience, hope, and a sense of well-being. By implementing the strategies and insights shared here, you can foster a positive outlook, celebrate small victories, and create a fulfilling life despite the challenges of CKD.

Remember, you are not alone in this journey. There is a wealth of resources, support networks, and healthcare professionals available to assist you. Let us embark on this journey together as we explore the path to wellness and empowerment with CKD.

# What is Chronic Kidney Disease (CKD)?

Chronic Kidney Disease (CKD) refers to a long-term condition characterized by the gradual loss of kidney function over time. It is a progressive condition in which the kidneys become damaged and are unable to perform their essential functions adequately.

The kidneys play a vital role in maintaining overall health by filtering waste products, excess fluid, and toxins from the blood, regulating electrolyte levels, and producing hormones that help control blood pressure and promote the production of red blood cells. In CKD, the kidneys' ability to carry out these functions becomes impaired.

CKD is typically diagnosed when kidney damage or decreased kidney function persists for three months or longer. It is often a result of underlying health conditions such as diabetes, high blood pressure, glomerulonephritis (inflammation of the kidney's filtering units), polycystic kidney disease (genetic disorder causing cysts in the kidneys), or other kidney-related disorders.

The severity of CKD is classified into stages based on the estimated glomerular filtration rate (eGFR), which measures how effectively the kidneys filter waste from the blood. The stages range from Stage 1 (mild kidney damage) to Stage 5 (end-stage renal disease or ESRD), where the kidneys are severely impaired, and dialysis or kidney transplantation becomes necessary for survival.

Managing chronic kidney disease involves various approaches, including lifestyle modifications (such as dietary changes and exercise), medications to control symptoms and manage underlying conditions, regular monitoring of kidney function, and in advanced cases, renal replacement therapy (dialysis or kidney transplantation). Early detection and intervention are crucial to slow down the progression of CKD and prevent complications associated with kidney failure.

It's important for individuals living with CKD to work closely with healthcare professionals, including nephrologists (kidney specialists), dietitians, and other members of the healthcare team, to develop a personalized treatment plan and make necessary lifestyle adjustments to promote kidney health and overall well-being.

# 1.2

# Understanding the Impact of CKD on Daily Life

Chronic Kidney Disease (CKD) can have a significant impact on daily life due to the essential role that kidneys play in maintaining overall health. As CKD progresses, it can lead to a range of physical, emotional, and lifestyle challenges that individuals with the condition must cope with. Some of the ways CKD can impact daily life include:

1. Fatigue and Weakness: As the kidneys become less efficient in filtering waste products and toxins from the blood, individuals with CKD may experience persistent fatigue

and weakness, making it challenging to carry out daily tasks and activities.

2. Fluid Retention and Swelling: CKD can lead to fluid retention in the body, causing swelling in the legs, ankles, and around the eyes. This swelling (edema) can be uncomfortable and may restrict mobility.

3. Changes in Urination: CKD can cause changes in urination patterns, including increased frequency or decreased output. This can disrupt sleep and daily routines.

4. Dietary Restrictions: People with CKD often need to adhere to strict dietary restrictions, limiting their intake of certain nutrients, especially sodium, potassium, and phosphorus. These restrictions can impact meal planning, dining out, and social activities involving food.

5. Increased Thirst: As the kidneys struggle to maintain fluid balance, individuals with CKD may experience excessive thirst, leading to increased water intake and frequent trips to the bathroom.

6. Anemia and Fatigue: CKD can lead to anemia, a condition characterized by a deficiency of red blood cells, resulting in fatigue, weakness, and difficulty concentrating.

7. Bone Health Issues: The kidneys play a role in maintaining calcium and phosphorus levels in the body. In CKD, imbalances can lead to bone health problems like osteoporosis or osteomalacia, increasing the risk of fractures.

8. High Blood Pressure: CKD and high blood pressure often go hand in hand. Uncontrolled

hypertension can further damage the kidneys and increase the risk of cardiovascular complications.

9. Emotional Impact: Dealing with a chronic condition can take a toll on a person's emotional well-being. Anxiety, depression, and stress are common emotional challenges faced by individuals with CKD.

10. Time Commitments: As CKD progresses, individuals may require regular medical appointments, laboratory tests, and treatments such as dialysis, which can demand significant time and energy.

11. Financial Strain: The cost of managing CKD, including medications, medical appointments, and treatments, can put a strain on an individual's finances.

Despite the challenges, with proper management and support, individuals living with CKD can lead fulfilling lives. Adhering to treatment plans, making lifestyle adjustments, seeking emotional support, and staying informed about the condition can all contribute to improving the overall quality of life for those with CKD. Regular communication with healthcare professionals is crucial for monitoring the condition's progress and making necessary adjustments to the treatment plan.

# 2.

# Stages of Chronic Kidney Disease

Chronic Kidney Disease (CKD) is typically categorized into five stages based on the estimated glomerular filtration rate (eGFR) and the presence of kidney damage. The stages of CKD help healthcare professionals determine the severity of the condition and guide treatment decisions. Here are the stages of CKD:

1. Stage 1: Kidney damage with normal or increased eGFR ($\geq 90$ ml/min/1.73m$^2$)

   - In this stage, there is evidence of kidney damage, such as abnormal urine tests or imaging studies, but the eGFR is still normal or only slightly decreased.

- People in Stage 1 CKD often have few or no symptoms, and kidney function is still relatively preserved.

2. Stage 2: Mild decrease in eGFR (60-89 ml/min/1.73m²)

   - In Stage 2, there is mild kidney damage with a slight decrease in the eGFR.

   - While symptoms may still be absent or minimal, there may be an increased risk of complications, and it becomes important to manage underlying conditions contributing to kidney damage, such as high blood pressure or diabetes.

3. Stage 3: Moderate decrease in eGFR (30-59 ml/min/1.73m²)

   - Stage 3 is further divided into two sub-stages: 3a (eGFR 45-59 ml/min/1.73m²) and 3b (eGFR 30-44 ml/min/1.73m²).

- Kidney function is noticeably reduced in Stage 3, and individuals may start experiencing symptoms like fatigue, fluid retention, and changes in urination patterns.

- Monitoring and management become crucial at this stage to slow down the progression of CKD and prevent complications.

4. Stage 4: Severe decrease in eGFR (15-29 ml/min/1.73m$^2$)

- Stage 4 is divided into two sub-stages: 4a (eGFR 15-29 ml/min/1.73m$^2$) and 4b (eGFR <15 ml/min/1.73m$^2$).

- At this stage, kidney function is significantly impaired, and individuals may experience symptoms like fatigue, anemia, bone problems, and increased risk of infections.

- Preparation for renal replacement therapy (dialysis or kidney transplantation) becomes necessary as kidney failure (Stage 5) approaches.

5. Stage 5: Kidney failure (eGFR <15 ml/min/1.73m² or requiring dialysis)

   - Also known as end-stage renal disease (ESRD), Stage 5 is characterized by a severe loss of kidney function.

   - Individuals in Stage 5 require renal replacement therapy, either through dialysis (hemodialysis or peritoneal dialysis) or kidney transplantation, to sustain life.

   - Symptoms are typically more severe at this stage, and close management by healthcare professionals is critical.


It's important to note that the progression of CKD can vary among individuals, and early detection and appropriate management can help slow down the progression, manage symptoms, and improve quality of life. Regular monitoring of kidney function, adherence to treatment plans, and lifestyle modifications play a crucial role in managing CKD at each stage.

# 3.

# Embracing Lifestyle Changes

Embracing lifestyle changes is an important aspect of managing Chronic Kidney Disease (CKD) and promoting overall well-being. These lifestyle modifications can help slow down the progression of CKD, manage symptoms, and reduce the risk of complications. Here are some key lifestyle changes that individuals with CKD can consider:

1. Diet and Nutrition:

   - Limit Sodium Intake: Reduce the consumption of processed foods, canned soups, and salty snacks, as high sodium levels can increase blood pressure and fluid retention.

- Control Protein Intake: Moderation is key. A dietitian can help determine the appropriate amount of protein to consume to minimize the strain on the kidneys.

- Manage Potassium and Phosphorus: Limit foods high in potassium and phosphorus, such as bananas, oranges, tomatoes, dairy products, and processed meats, as the kidneys may have difficulty processing these minerals.

- Maintain a Healthy Weight: Achieving and maintaining a healthy weight through balanced nutrition can help manage blood pressure and improve overall health.

2. Hydration:

- Ensure Adequate Fluid Intake: Drink enough fluids as recommended by a healthcare professional to maintain proper hydration, but be mindful of any fluid restrictions based on individual circumstances.

3. Exercise and Physical Activity:

   - Engage in Regular Physical Activity: Regular exercise can help manage weight, lower blood pressure, improve cardiovascular health, and enhance overall well-being. Consult with a healthcare professional before starting or modifying an exercise routine.

4. Medication Adherence:

   - Take Medications as Prescribed: Adhere to the prescribed medications and follow the recommended dosage schedule. Medications may include those for blood pressure control, anemia management, and phosphate binders, among others.

5. Smoking Cessation:

   - Quit Smoking: Smoking can further damage blood vessels and worsen kidney function.

Quitting smoking can have numerous health benefits.

6. Stress Management:

   - Adopt Stress-Reduction Techniques: Practice stress management techniques such as deep breathing exercises, meditation, yoga, or engaging in hobbies or activities that promote relaxation and well-being.

7. Regular Monitoring and Follow-up:

   - Attend Medical Appointments: Regularly visit healthcare professionals to monitor kidney function, adjust treatment plans, and address any concerns or questions.

8. Support System:

   - Seek Support from Family, Friends, and Support Groups: Building a strong support system can provide emotional support, motivation, and understanding during the CKD journey.

It's crucial to work closely with healthcare professionals, including nephrologists and dietitians, to develop an individualized plan tailored to specific needs and stage of CKD. Adapting to lifestyle changes can take time, and it's important to approach them gradually and seek professional guidance throughout the process.

# 3.1

# Managing Diet and Nutrition for Kidney Health

Managing diet and nutrition is essential for maintaining kidney health and managing Chronic Kidney Disease (CKD). A well-planned diet can help slow down the progression of CKD, control symptoms, and reduce the risk of complications. Here are some key considerations for managing diet and nutrition for kidney health:

1. Sodium (Salt) Intake:

   - Limit Sodium: Reduce the consumption of processed and packaged foods, canned soups, salty snacks, and fast food, as they are often high in sodium. Aim to stay within the recommended daily sodium intake as advised by a healthcare professional.

2. Protein Intake:

   - Moderate Protein Consumption: Work with a registered dietitian to determine the appropriate amount of protein for your stage of CKD. Moderation is key to avoid putting excess strain on the kidneys. High-quality protein sources like lean meats, poultry, fish, eggs, and dairy products are generally recommended.

3. Potassium and Phosphorus Management:

   - Monitor Potassium Intake: Limit high-potassium foods such as bananas, oranges, tomatoes, potatoes, spinach, and beans, as elevated potassium levels can be harmful to the kidneys. Your dietitian can help create a personalized plan based on your specific needs.

   - Control Phosphorus Intake: Limit phosphorus-rich foods like dairy products, processed meats, carbonated drinks, and certain whole grains. Phosphate binders may also be prescribed to help control phosphorus levels.

4. Fluid Intake:

   - Follow Fluid Recommendations: Maintain an appropriate fluid balance as advised by your healthcare professional. In advanced stages of CKD, fluid restrictions may be necessary to avoid fluid overload and swelling. Monitor and adjust fluid intake based on individual circumstances and recommendations.

5. Healthy Weight and Caloric Intake:

   - Achieve and Maintain a Healthy Weight: Maintain a balanced diet and monitor portion sizes to manage weight. Excess weight can increase the risk of complications and put additional strain on the kidneys.

- Consult with a dietitian or healthcare professional to determine the appropriate caloric intake based on your age, gender, weight, activity level, and overall health goals.

6. Phosphate Binders and Medication:

   - Take Medications as Prescribed: If prescribed phosphate binders or other medications to manage specific aspects of kidney disease, follow the prescribed dosage and timing guidelines.

7. Considerations for Individualized Diet Plans:

   - Individualized Plans: Work with a registered dietitian who specializes in kidney health to develop a personalized meal plan that suits your specific needs, taking into account your stage of CKD, underlying conditions, medications, and personal preferences.

- Monitor and Adjust: Regularly monitor lab results and kidney function, and consult with your dietitian to make necessary adjustments to your diet plan.

Remember, managing diet and nutrition for kidney health is highly individualized, and it's important to work closely with healthcare professionals, particularly registered dietitians or renal dietitians, who can provide specialized guidance and support. They can help develop a meal plan that balances nutritional needs, manages CKD-related concerns, and supports overall well-being.

Here's a sample one-week meal plan for a patient with Chronic Kidney Disease (CKD). Please note that this is a general meal plan, and individualized recommendations may vary depending on the specific needs, stage of CKD, and other factors. It's important to consult with a registered dietitian or healthcare professional for personalized advice.

Day 1:

- Breakfast: Vegetable omelet made with egg whites, spinach, and onions. Whole grain toast with a small amount of margarine. Fresh berries.

- Snack: Carrot sticks with a side of hummus.

- Lunch: Grilled chicken breast, steamed broccoli, and quinoa.

- Snack: Greek yogurt with low-potassium fruits like sliced apples.

- Dinner: Baked salmon, roasted asparagus, brown rice, and a mixed green salad with lemon juice and olive oil dressing.

- Snack: Air-popped popcorn.

Day 2:

- Breakfast: Oatmeal made with water, topped with sliced banana and a sprinkle of cinnamon. Herbal tea.

- Snack: Low-phosphorus protein bar.

- Lunch: Turkey lettuce wraps with low-sodium turkey breast, lettuce, and diced tomatoes. Side of cucumber and tomato salad.

- Snack: Rice cakes with almond butter.

- Dinner: Grilled shrimp skewers, steamed green beans, wild rice, and a side salad with low-potassium vegetables.

- Snack: Sugar-free gelatin.


Day 3:

- Breakfast: Whole grain toast with mashed avocado and sliced tomatoes. Fresh fruit salad.

- Snack: Handful of unsalted almonds.

- Lunch: Quinoa and black bean salad with diced bell peppers and cilantro.

- Snack: Low-fat cottage cheese with sliced peaches.

- Dinner: Baked chicken breast, roasted Brussels sprouts, sweet potato mash.

- Snack: Rice crackers with low-sodium salsa.


Day 4:

- Breakfast: Vegetable and cheese omelet made with egg whites, bell peppers, and low-potassium cheese. Whole grain toast.

- Snack: Celery sticks with peanut butter.

- Lunch: Grilled tofu, stir-fried mixed vegetables, and brown rice.

- Snack: Low-fat yogurt with a sprinkle of ground flaxseed.

- Dinner: Baked white fish, steamed cauliflower, quinoa pilaf.

- Snack: Carrot cake energy balls (made with shredded carrots, oats, and nuts).

Day 5:

- Breakfast: Buckwheat pancakes with sugar-free syrup and sliced strawberries. Herbal tea.

- Snack: Rice cakes with guacamole.

- Lunch: Lentil soup with a side of mixed greens.

- Snack: Low-potassium fruit smoothie made with almond milk.

- Dinner: Grilled lean beef, roasted zucchini, mashed potatoes (moderate portion).

- Snack: Air-popped popcorn.


Day 6:

- Breakfast: Spinach and feta cheese scramble made with egg whites. Whole grain toast with a small amount of margarine. Fresh melon.

- Snack: Greek yogurt with sliced almonds.

- Lunch: Chicken and vegetable stir-fry with low-sodium sauce, served over brown rice.

- Snack: Rice cakes with low-sodium peanut butter.

- Dinner: Baked cod, steamed asparagus, wild rice.

- Snack: Sugar-free gelatin.


Day 7:

- Breakfast: Vegetable and cheese frittata made with egg whites, spinach, and low-potassium cheese. Whole grain toast.

- Snack: Carrot sticks with hummus.

- Lunch: Quinoa salad with cherry tomatoes, cucumber, and diced chicken breast.

- Snack: Low-fat cottage cheese with mixed berries.

- Dinner: Grilled

It's important to note that a meal plan for a patient with Chronic Kidney Disease (CKD) should be individualized based on their specific needs, stage of CKD, lab results, medications, and any other underlying health conditions. However, here is a general overview of a CKD-friendly meal plan:

Breakfast:

- Egg white omelet with vegetables (such as spinach, bell peppers, and onions)

- Whole grain toast with a small amount of margarine or avocado

- Fresh fruit (such as berries or apple slices)

- Herbal tea or water

Snack:

- A small handful of unsalted almonds or a low-phosphorus protein bar

- Carrot sticks or cucumber slices

Lunch:

- Grilled chicken breast or fish (such as salmon or tilapia)

- Steamed or roasted vegetables (such as broccoli, cauliflower, or asparagus)

- Quinoa or brown rice

- Mixed green salad with low-potassium vegetables (such as lettuce, cucumbers, and radishes) dressed with lemon juice and olive oil

Snack:

- Low-potassium fruits, like apples or grapes

- Greek yogurt (low-fat or non-fat) or a small serving of cottage cheese

Dinner:

- Baked or grilled lean meat (chicken, turkey, or lean beef)

- Steamed or sautéed low-potassium vegetables (such as green beans, zucchini, or mushrooms)

- Whole wheat pasta or couscous

- Fresh salad with low-potassium ingredients and a vinegar-based dressing


Snack (if needed):

- Air-popped popcorn or rice cakes

- Sugar-free gelatin or a small portion of low-potassium dessert


Fluids:

- Follow the fluid recommendations given by your healthcare professional. This can vary depending on your stage of CKD and individual needs.

It's important to work with a registered dietitian who specializes in kidney health to tailor a meal plan that meets your specific dietary requirements. They can provide detailed guidance on portion sizes, food choices, and strategies to manage sodium, potassium, phosphorus, and protein intake based on your individual needs and preferences.

Remember, this is a general meal plan, and it's crucial to consult with your healthcare team for personalized advice and to make adjustments based on your specific dietary needs and lab results.

# 3.2

# Importance of Hydration and Fluid Intake

Hydration and fluid intake are crucial aspects of maintaining overall health, and they play a particularly significant role in managing Chronic Kidney Disease (CKD). Here are some key points highlighting the importance of hydration and fluid intake:

1. Kidney Function: Adequate hydration is essential for supporting optimal kidney function. The kidneys filter waste products and toxins from the bloodstream, and sufficient fluid intake helps facilitate this process. It promotes urine production, which helps remove waste and maintain electrolyte balance.

2. Blood Pressure Control: Proper hydration helps regulate blood pressure. When the body is dehydrated, blood volume decreases, leading to increased blood pressure. In individuals with CKD, high blood pressure can further damage the kidneys, so maintaining adequate hydration is important for blood pressure management.

3. Fluid Balance: Maintaining the right balance of fluids is crucial for individuals with CKD, especially in advanced stages of the disease. Fluid restrictions may be necessary to prevent fluid overload, swelling (edema), and other complications. On the other hand, dehydration should be avoided, as it can lead to complications like electrolyte imbalances and decreased kidney function.

4. Toxin Removal: Sufficient fluid intake helps dilute and eliminate waste products and toxins from the body through urine. This is

particularly important for individuals with compromised kidney function, as impaired kidneys may struggle to effectively filter waste without proper hydration.

5. Electrolyte Balance: Adequate hydration helps maintain electrolyte balance in the body, which is crucial for normal cell function, nerve transmission, and muscle contractions. Electrolytes like sodium, potassium, and chloride need to be properly regulated, and adequate fluid intake supports this balance.

6. Prevention of Kidney Stones: Staying hydrated is one of the key strategies for preventing kidney stones. Sufficient water intake helps dilute urine and reduces the risk of crystal formation and stone development in the kidneys.

7. Management of Urinary Tract Infections (UTIs): Drinking enough fluids can help flush bacteria out of the urinary tract and prevent UTIs. UTIs can be more common in individuals with CKD and can lead to complications if not promptly treated.

It's important to note that fluid needs can vary depending on individual factors, such as stage of CKD, presence of other health conditions, and any fluid restrictions prescribed by a healthcare professional. It's recommended to consult with a healthcare team, including nephrologists and dietitians, to determine the appropriate fluid intake for individual circumstances.

Remember, maintaining proper hydration and fluid intake is crucial for kidney health, but it's equally important to follow any fluid restrictions or recommendations provided by your healthcare team to manage CKD effectively.

# 3.3

# Incorporating Exercise into Daily Routine

Incorporating exercise into your daily routine is beneficial for overall health and can be particularly advantageous for individuals living with Chronic Kidney Disease (CKD). Regular physical activity can help improve cardiovascular fitness, maintain a healthy weight, manage blood pressure, enhance mood, and increase overall well-being. Here are some tips for incorporating exercise into your daily routine:

1. Consult with Your Healthcare Team: Before starting or modifying an exercise program, consult with your healthcare team, including

your nephrologist or healthcare provider. They can provide guidance and recommendations tailored to your specific condition and stage of CKD.

2. Choose Low-Impact Activities: Opt for low-impact exercises that are easier on the joints and less likely to cause injury. Examples include walking, cycling, swimming, water aerobics, tai chi, and yoga. These activities provide cardiovascular benefits without putting excessive strain on the kidneys or other body systems.

3. Start Slowly and Gradually Increase Intensity: If you're new to exercise or have been inactive for a while, start with low-intensity activities and gradually increase the duration and intensity over time. This gradual approach helps reduce the risk of injury and allows your body to adapt to the demands of exercise.

4. Set Realistic Goals: Set realistic goals based on your fitness level and health condition. Start with small, achievable targets and gradually work your way up. Remember that consistency is key, and even short bouts of exercise can be beneficial.

5. Incorporate Strength Training: Include strength training exercises at least two days a week. These exercises can help improve muscle strength, endurance, and bone health. Use light weights, resistance bands, or bodyweight exercises such as squats, lunges, and push-ups. Work with a qualified fitness professional to ensure proper form and technique.

6. Listen to Your Body: Pay attention to how your body responds to exercise. If you experience pain, shortness of breath, dizziness,

or other concerning symptoms, stop exercising and consult with your healthcare provider.

7. Stay Hydrated: Drink water before, during, and after exercise to stay hydrated. Proper hydration is important for kidney health and overall well-being.

8. Warm-Up and Cool-Down: Before starting your exercise routine, warm up your muscles with gentle movements and stretches. Afterward, cool down with light stretching to promote flexibility and prevent muscle soreness.

9. Find Activities You Enjoy: Choose activities that you enjoy and that fit your lifestyle. This increases the likelihood of sticking to your exercise routine and makes it more enjoyable.

10. Stay Consistent: Aim for regular exercise sessions throughout the week. Even if you have busy days, find opportunities to be active, such as taking short walks during breaks or parking farther away from your destination to increase your daily steps.

Remember, it's important to work with your healthcare team to determine the most suitable exercise program for your specific condition. They can provide personalized recommendations and monitor your progress along the way.

# 3.4

# Stress Management and Mental Health Support

Stress management and mental health support are crucial aspects of overall well-being, particularly for individuals living with Chronic Kidney Disease (CKD). Coping with the challenges of CKD, such as lifestyle adjustments, treatment plans, and potential complications, can cause emotional and psychological stress. Here are some strategies for managing stress and seeking mental health support:

1. Seek Emotional Support: Reach out to your support system, including family, friends, and loved ones, to share your feelings and

experiences. They can provide understanding, empathy, and a listening ear. Joining support groups for individuals with CKD can also connect you with others facing similar challenges and provide a sense of community.

2. Consult with Mental Health Professionals: Consider consulting with mental health professionals, such as therapists, psychologists, or counselors, who specialize in chronic illness or kidney-related issues. They can help you develop coping strategies, provide emotional support, and assist in managing anxiety, depression, or other mental health concerns.

3. Practice Stress-Relieving Techniques:

   - Deep Breathing: Practice deep breathing exercises to help calm your mind and body. Focus on slow, deep breaths, inhaling deeply through your nose and exhaling through your mouth.

   - Meditation and Mindfulness: Engage in meditation or mindfulness practices to promote relaxation and reduce stress. This involves focusing your attention on the present moment, observing your thoughts and emotions without judgment.

   - Relaxation Techniques: Explore relaxation techniques like progressive muscle relaxation, guided imagery, or listening to soothing music to alleviate stress and promote a sense of calm.

4. Physical Activity: Engage in regular physical activity as it can help reduce stress and improve mood. Choose activities that you enjoy and are appropriate for your fitness level and health condition. Exercise releases endorphins, which are natural mood enhancers.

5. Prioritize Self-Care: Take time for self-care activities that bring you joy and relaxation. This could include hobbies, reading, spending time in nature, taking warm baths, practicing yoga, or engaging in creative outlets. It's important to allocate time for activities that help you recharge and rejuvenate.

6. Maintain a Healthy Lifestyle: Adopting a healthy lifestyle can positively impact your mental health. This includes getting adequate sleep, eating a balanced diet, limiting caffeine and alcohol intake, and avoiding smoking or illicit drug use. These lifestyle factors contribute to overall well-being and can help manage stress levels.

7. Communicate with Your Healthcare Team: Be open and honest with your healthcare team about your mental health concerns. They can

provide guidance, refer you to appropriate resources, and collaborate with mental health professionals to ensure holistic care.

Remember, seeking mental health support is not a sign of weakness but a proactive step toward maintaining your overall well-being. Your mental health is as important as your physical health, and addressing stress and emotional concerns can positively impact your ability to manage CKD effectively.

# 4.

# Medications and Treatment Options

The treatment of Chronic Kidney Disease (CKD) involves a combination of lifestyle modifications, medication management, and sometimes advanced medical interventions. Here are some common medications and treatment options used in the management of CKD:

1. Blood Pressure Medications: High blood pressure is a common complication of CKD. Medications like angiotensin-converting enzyme (ACE) inhibitors and angiotensin receptor blockers (ARBs) are commonly prescribed to help control blood pressure and protect the kidneys from further damage.

2. Medications for Proteinuria: Proteinuria, or the presence of excess protein in the urine, is another common complication of CKD. Medications like angiotensin receptor blockers (ARBs) and angiotensin-converting enzyme (ACE) inhibitors are often used to reduce proteinuria and slow the progression of kidney damage.

3. Diuretics: Diuretics help promote urine production and can be prescribed to manage fluid retention and control blood pressure in individuals with CKD.

4. Phosphate Binders: For individuals with advanced CKD or end-stage renal disease (ESRD), phosphate binders may be prescribed to control high levels of phosphate in the blood. These medications bind to dietary

phosphate and prevent its absorption in the gut, reducing phosphate levels.

5. Erythropoiesis-Stimulating Agents (ESAs): In cases of anemia associated with CKD, erythropoiesis-stimulating agents may be prescribed to stimulate the production of red blood cells and improve hemoglobin levels.

6. Iron Supplements: Iron deficiency is common in individuals with CKD. Iron supplements may be prescribed to address iron deficiency anemia and support the production of healthy red blood cells.

7. Dietary Modifications: Along with medications, dietary modifications play a critical role in managing CKD. A diet low in sodium, phosphorus, and potassium, and potentially limited in protein, may be

recommended to help manage fluid balance, blood pressure, and electrolyte levels.

8. Dialysis: For individuals with advanced CKD or ESRD, dialysis may be necessary. Dialysis is a medical procedure that removes waste products, excess fluids, and toxins from the blood when the kidneys can no longer adequately perform these functions.

9. Kidney Transplant: In some cases of advanced CKD or ESRD, a kidney transplant may be an option. This involves surgically replacing the failed kidney with a healthy kidney from a living or deceased donor.

It's important to note that the choice of medication and treatment options depends on various factors, including the individual's stage of CKD, overall health, and specific needs. The treatment plan is typically developed by a healthcare team, including nephrologists, dietitians, and other specialists, who work together to provide personalized care based on individual circumstances.

It's crucial to follow the treatment plan prescribed by your healthcare team, take medications as prescribed, and attend regular medical appointments to monitor your kidney function and overall health.

# 4.1

# Understanding Medications for CKD

Understanding the medications used in the treatment of Chronic Kidney Disease (CKD) can help individuals manage their condition effectively. Here are some important points to consider:

1. Blood Pressure Medications: Controlling high blood pressure is crucial in managing CKD. Medications like angiotensin-converting enzyme (ACE) inhibitors and angiotensin receptor blockers (ARBs) are commonly prescribed. They help relax blood vessels, lower blood pressure, and protect the kidneys from further damage.

2. Medications for Proteinuria: Proteinuria, the presence of excess protein in the urine, is a sign of kidney damage. Medications like ACE inhibitors and ARBs can be used to reduce proteinuria and slow down the progression of CKD.

3. Diuretics: Diuretics are medications that increase urine production and help manage fluid retention. They are often prescribed to control blood pressure and reduce edema (swelling) in individuals with CKD.

4. Phosphate Binders: In advanced stages of CKD, the kidneys may have difficulty removing excess phosphate from the body. High phosphate levels can lead to complications. Phosphate binders are medications that bind to dietary phosphate in the gut, preventing its absorption and reducing phosphate levels in the blood.

5. Erythropoiesis-Stimulating Agents (ESAs): CKD can cause anemia due to decreased production of red blood cells. ESAs are medications that stimulate the bone marrow to produce more red blood cells, improving anemia and reducing fatigue.

6. Iron Supplements: Iron deficiency is common in CKD and can contribute to anemia. Iron supplements may be prescribed to address iron deficiency and support the production of healthy red blood cells.

7. Statins: Individuals with CKD are at an increased risk of cardiovascular disease. Statins are cholesterol-lowering medications that may be prescribed to manage high cholesterol levels and reduce the risk of heart disease.

8. Anticoagulants: In some cases, individuals with CKD may require anticoagulant medications to prevent the formation of blood clots or to manage certain cardiovascular conditions.

9. Medications for Symptom Management: Depending on individual symptoms and complications, other medications may be prescribed. For example, medications for managing pain, itching, nausea, or managing specific kidney-related conditions like urinary tract infections (UTIs) or kidney stones.

It's essential to follow the prescribed medication regimen, take medications as directed by healthcare professionals, and inform them of any side effects or concerns. Regular communication with your healthcare team, including nephrologists and pharmacists, is important to ensure that medications are properly managed and adjusted as needed.

It's also important to note that medication requirements may vary depending on an individual's stage of CKD, overall health, and the presence of other conditions or medications. Healthcare professionals will consider these factors and tailor the treatment plan to meet individual needs.

## 4.2

# Dialysis: Types and Considerations

Dialysis is a medical procedure used to perform the functions of the kidneys when they are no longer able to adequately filter waste products and excess fluid from the blood. There are two main types of dialysis: hemodialysis and peritoneal dialysis. Here's an overview of each type and some considerations associated with dialysis:

1. Hemodialysis:

   - Procedure: Hemodialysis involves filtering the blood outside the body using a machine called a dialyzer or artificial kidney. Blood is drawn from a vascular access point (typically an arteriovenous fistula or graft) and circulated through the dialyzer, where it is cleansed before being returned to the body.

- Treatment Frequency: Hemodialysis is typically performed in a dialysis center or hospital setting, usually three times a week, with each session lasting several hours.

- Vascular Access: Creating a suitable vascular access is an important consideration for hemodialysis. This involves surgically connecting an artery and vein to create a site where blood can be easily accessed for dialysis.

- Dietary Restrictions: Hemodialysis patients often have dietary restrictions, particularly regarding fluid intake, sodium, potassium, and phosphorus. This is to help maintain fluid and electrolyte balance in the body.

- Lifestyle Impact: Hemodialysis treatments require regular visits to the dialysis center and can have an impact on daily activities and scheduling.

2. Peritoneal Dialysis:

- Procedure: Peritoneal dialysis uses the lining of the abdomen, called the peritoneum, as a natural filter. A dialysis solution (dialysate) is introduced into the abdomen through a catheter, and waste products and excess fluid pass from the bloodstream through the peritoneum into the dialysate. After a set dwell time, the used dialysate is drained out of the abdomen and replaced with fresh dialysate.

- Treatment Frequency: Peritoneal dialysis is typically performed at home and can be done daily, including during the night using a machine called a cycler, or manually through regular exchanges throughout the day.

- Catheter Placement: The placement of a peritoneal dialysis catheter is necessary for the procedure. It is inserted through a small incision in the abdomen and positioned in the peritoneal cavity.

- Peritoneal Catheter Care: Proper care and hygiene are important for maintaining the health and function of the peritoneal dialysis catheter, including regular dressing changes and preventing infection.

- Dietary Considerations: Peritoneal dialysis may provide more flexibility with dietary choices compared to hemodialysis, although dietary restrictions may still be necessary depending on individual needs.

Considerations for Dialysis:

- Access to Care: Access to a dialysis center, specialized healthcare professionals, and necessary equipment is crucial for successful dialysis treatment.

- Lifestyle Impact: Both hemodialysis and peritoneal dialysis have implications on a person's lifestyle and daily routine. Consider the impact on work, travel, and other activities when choosing the appropriate type of dialysis.

- Emotional and Psychological Support: Dialysis can be emotionally and psychologically challenging. Seek support from healthcare providers, support groups, and loved ones to help manage the emotional aspects of living with dialysis.

- Long-Term Planning: Depending on the individual's condition, dialysis may be a temporary or long-term treatment option. For those considering kidney transplantation, discussions with healthcare providers about eligibility and the transplantation process are important.

# 4.3

# Kidney Transplantation: When and How?

Kidney transplantation is considered when an individual's kidney function has deteriorated to the point where dialysis is no longer sufficient or desirable. Here's some information on when and how kidney transplantation is performed:

When is Kidney Transplantation Considered?

1. Advanced Stage of CKD: Kidney transplantation is typically considered when an individual reaches the advanced stages of Chronic Kidney Disease (CKD) or End-Stage Renal Disease (ESRD). This is when kidney function has significantly declined, and the individual's quality of life and overall health are compromised.

2. Dialysis-Dependent: Kidney transplantation may be considered for individuals who are dependent on dialysis for an extended period. While dialysis helps replace kidney function, a kidney transplant offers the potential for a more normal and improved quality of life.

3. Health Evaluation: Candidates for kidney transplantation undergo a thorough evaluation process to assess their overall health and suitability for the procedure. This evaluation involves various medical tests, including blood tests, imaging studies, and consultations with a transplant team that includes nephrologists, surgeons, psychologists, and other specialists.

How is Kidney Transplantation Performed?

1. Donor Options: Kidneys for transplantation can come from two main sources: living donors and deceased donors.

- Living Donors: A living donor is typically a family member, friend, or willing individual who volunteers to donate one of their healthy kidneys. Living donor transplants often provide better outcomes due to the availability of a healthy organ and reduced waiting time.

- Deceased Donors: Deceased donor kidneys come from individuals who have agreed to donate their organs upon their death. These kidneys are matched to potential recipients based on factors such as blood type, tissue compatibility, and waiting time on the transplant list.


2. Transplant Procedure: The kidney transplant surgery involves removing the diseased kidney(s) and implanting the healthy donor kidney(s) in the recipient. The transplanted kidney is usually placed in the lower abdomen, and the blood vessels and ureter (tube that carries urine) are connected to the recipient's blood vessels and bladder.

3. Post-Transplant Care: After the transplant surgery, individuals will require ongoing medical care and close monitoring to ensure the success of the transplant. This includes taking immunosuppressant medications to prevent rejection of the transplanted kidney. Regular follow-up visits with the transplant team are necessary to monitor kidney function, adjust medications, and address any potential complications.

4. Lifelong Commitment: Kidney transplantation is not a cure for CKD, but it offers an opportunity for improved quality of life and increased longevity compared to dialysis. It's important to note that transplant recipients will need to adhere to lifelong medication regimens, follow a healthy lifestyle, and regularly visit their healthcare providers for monitoring and care.

The decision to pursue kidney transplantation is a complex one that involves careful consideration of individual factors, including overall health, suitability for surgery, availability of a compatible donor, and the potential benefits and risks. It's crucial to have thorough discussions with healthcare providers, transplant teams, and loved ones to make an informed decision and receive the necessary support throughout the process.

# 5.1

# Dealing with Fatigue and Sleep Issues

Living with Chronic Kidney Disease (CKD) can present various challenges and potential complications. Here are some common challenges individuals may face and strategies for navigating them:

1. Fatigue and Weakness: CKD can cause fatigue and weakness due to anemia, fluid imbalances, and the buildup of waste products in the body. It's important to prioritize rest, maintain a balanced diet, manage fluid intake, and follow the prescribed treatment plan, including taking medications to manage anemia or other related symptoms.

2. Dietary Restrictions: CKD often requires dietary modifications, including restrictions on sodium, potassium, phosphorus, and protein intake. Working with a registered dietitian who specializes in kidney disease can help create a personalized meal plan that meets nutritional needs while managing CKD. Compliance with dietary restrictions can help maintain fluid and electrolyte balance and prevent complications.

3. Emotional and Psychological Impact: Living with a chronic illness like CKD can have emotional and psychological effects. It's essential to seek emotional support from healthcare professionals, support groups, or therapists to cope with feelings of stress, anxiety, or depression. Engaging in relaxation techniques, hobbies, and maintaining a strong support system can also contribute to mental well-being.

4. Financial Considerations: Managing CKD and its treatments can be costly. It's important to understand insurance coverage, explore financial assistance programs, and communicate with healthcare providers about any financial concerns. Seeking financial counseling or support from patient advocacy groups may also be helpful.

5. Medication Management: Keeping track of multiple medications and their schedules can be challenging. Establishing a medication routine, using pill organizers, and setting reminders can help ensure timely and accurate medication administration. Regularly communicating with healthcare providers about any difficulties or concerns with medications is crucial.

6. Fluid and Weight Management: Maintaining fluid balance is vital in CKD management. Monitoring and controlling fluid intake as

advised by healthcare professionals can help prevent fluid overload and associated complications. Regularly monitoring weight can also be an essential indicator of fluid balance.

7. Infections and Immune Health: Individuals with CKD may be more susceptible to infections due to compromised immune function. Following good hygiene practices, receiving recommended vaccinations, and promptly seeking medical attention for any signs of infection are important for maintaining overall health.

8. Cardiovascular Health: CKD increases the risk of cardiovascular diseases. It's important to manage blood pressure, cholesterol levels, and blood sugar levels through lifestyle modifications, medications, and regular monitoring. Engaging in regular physical

activity, as permitted by healthcare providers, can also support cardiovascular health.

9. Regular Medical Follow-up: Regular medical check-ups and follow-up appointments with healthcare providers, including nephrologists and other specialists, are essential for monitoring kidney function, managing complications, adjusting treatment plans, and addressing any concerns.

Navigating the challenges and potential complications of CKD requires a multidisciplinary approach involving healthcare professionals, family support, and self-care. Open communication, adherence to treatment plans, and proactive management of lifestyle factors can help individuals with CKD lead fulfilling lives and optimize their overall well-being.

# 5.2
# Handling Anemia and Bone Health

Fatigue and sleep issues are common challenges for individuals living with Chronic Kidney Disease (CKD). Here are some strategies that can help in dealing with these issues:

1. Prioritize Rest and Sleep: Ensure you are getting enough rest and prioritize sleep. Aim for a regular sleep schedule and create a comfortable sleep environment that promotes relaxation and quality sleep.

2. Manage Anemia: Anemia, a common complication of CKD, can contribute to fatigue. Work with your healthcare provider to monitor and manage your hemoglobin levels. They may prescribe medications such as erythropoiesis-stimulating agents (ESAs) or iron supplements to help boost red blood cell production and alleviate anemia-related fatigue.

3. Follow a Balanced Diet: Proper nutrition plays a crucial role in managing fatigue. Follow the dietary recommendations provided by your healthcare team, including consuming an appropriate amount of calories, protein, and other essential nutrients. A registered dietitian with expertise in kidney disease can help create a meal plan that meets your specific needs.

4. Manage Fluid Intake: Maintaining a proper balance of fluids is important for overall health and can help alleviate sleep disruptions caused

by excessive nighttime urination. Work with your healthcare provider or a registered dietitian to determine the appropriate daily fluid intake for your condition and adhere to it.

5. Regular Physical Activity: Engaging in regular physical activity, as recommended by your healthcare provider, can improve energy levels and overall well-being. Choose activities that are suitable for your fitness level and health condition. Even light exercise, such as walking, can help combat fatigue.

6. Stress Management Techniques: Stress can contribute to fatigue and disrupt sleep patterns. Explore stress management techniques such as deep breathing exercises, meditation, yoga, or engaging in activities that you find relaxing and enjoyable. Consult with a mental health professional if stress becomes overwhelming.

7. Monitor Medications: Some medications used to manage CKD and related conditions can cause fatigue or sleep disturbances as side effects. If you suspect that a specific medication is affecting your energy levels or sleep, discuss it with your healthcare provider to explore alternative options or adjust the dosage.

8. Seek Emotional Support: Living with a chronic illness can be emotionally challenging. Seek support from family, friends, support groups, or mental health professionals who can provide guidance and help you cope with fatigue and sleep issues.

9. Communicate with Your Healthcare Team: Regularly communicate with your healthcare team about your fatigue and sleep issues. They can help identify any underlying causes, make

necessary adjustments to your treatment plan, and provide additional support or referrals as needed.

Remember, everyone's experience with fatigue and sleep issues may vary, and it's important to tailor strategies to your individual needs. Working closely with your healthcare team and maintaining open communication can help in finding the most effective solutions for managing fatigue and improving sleep quality.

Anemia and bone health are important considerations for individuals living with Chronic Kidney Disease (CKD). Here are some strategies for handling anemia and promoting bone health:

1. Managing Anemia:

   - Medications: Your healthcare provider may prescribe erythropoiesis-stimulating agents (ESAs) or iron supplements to stimulate red blood cell production and manage anemia. It's important to take these medications as prescribed and undergo regular monitoring of hemoglobin levels.

  - Iron-rich Diet: Incorporate iron-rich foods into your diet, such as lean meats, poultry, fish, legumes, dark leafy greens, and fortified cereals. Vitamin C-rich foods, like citrus fruits, can enhance iron absorption.

  - Avoid Phosphorus Binders: Some phosphorus binders used to manage phosphorus levels in CKD can interfere with iron absorption. Discuss this with your healthcare provider to ensure the appropriate timing and administration of medications.

2. Promoting Bone Health:

  - Calcium Intake: Consume an adequate amount of calcium through dietary sources such as low-fat dairy products, fortified plant-based milk, calcium-rich vegetables (e.g., broccoli, kale), and calcium supplements if recommended by your healthcare provider. Aim for the appropriate daily calcium intake for your age and gender.

  - Vitamin D: Vitamin D plays a crucial role in calcium absorption and bone health. Ensure sufficient vitamin D levels through sun exposure and/or supplementation as advised by your healthcare provider.

  - Phosphorus Management: Excessive phosphorus levels can lead to bone problems. Limit phosphorus intake by avoiding high-phosphorus foods, including processed meats, carbonated beverages, and certain processed foods. Take phosphorus binders as prescribed to control phosphorus levels.

  - Regular Exercise: Engage in weight-bearing exercises, such as walking or light resistance training, as recommended by your healthcare provider. These exercises help improve bone density and strength.

- Quit Smoking: Smoking can increase the risk of bone loss. If you smoke, consider quitting to protect your bone health.

- Monitor Bone Mineral Density (BMD): Your healthcare provider may periodically assess your bone health through a bone density test (DEXA scan). Regular monitoring helps identify any changes or potential issues.

3. Work with a Healthcare Team:

- Regularly communicate with your healthcare team, including nephrologists, dietitians, and other specialists, to monitor and manage anemia and bone health. They can provide guidance, adjust medications, and offer personalized recommendations based on your specific needs.

It's important to note that the management of anemia and bone health may vary depending on the stage of CKD, individual needs, and specific recommendations from your healthcare provider. Following their guidance, adhering to the prescribed treatment plan, and maintaining open communication are crucial in handling anemia and promoting optimal bone health.

# 5.3

# Managing Hypertension and Cardiovascular Health

Managing hypertension and cardiovascular health is crucial for individuals with Chronic Kidney Disease (CKD). Here are some strategies to help in this regard:

1. Blood Pressure Control:

- Medications: Work with your healthcare provider to identify appropriate medications to control hypertension. Commonly prescribed medications include ACE inhibitors, angiotensin II receptor blockers (ARBs), diuretics, and calcium channel blockers. Adhere to the prescribed medication regimen and attend regular follow-up appointments for blood pressure monitoring.

- Sodium Restriction: Limit your sodium intake by avoiding processed and packaged foods, fast food, and excessive salt use during cooking. Instead, use herbs, spices, and salt alternatives to enhance the flavor of your meals.

- Dietary Approaches to Stop Hypertension (DASH): Follow the DASH diet, which emphasizes fruits, vegetables, whole grains, lean proteins, and low-fat dairy products. This dietary approach has been shown to lower blood pressure and improve cardiovascular health.

- Weight Management: Maintain a healthy weight or work toward achieving a healthy weight through a combination of a balanced diet and regular physical activity. Weight loss, if needed, can help reduce blood pressure.

2. Cardiovascular Health Promotion:

- Cholesterol Control: Monitor and manage your cholesterol levels through dietary modifications, regular exercise, and medication if necessary. Limit saturated and trans fats in your diet and include heart-healthy fats like omega-3 fatty acids found in fish, nuts, and seeds.

- Blood Sugar Management: If you have diabetes in addition to CKD, it's important to manage your blood sugar levels as high blood sugar can contribute to cardiovascular complications. Follow your prescribed treatment plan, including medications, dietary recommendations, and blood sugar monitoring.

- Smoking Cessation: Quit smoking if you smoke. Smoking is a significant risk factor for cardiovascular disease. Seek support from healthcare professionals, support groups, or smoking cessation programs to quit smoking successfully.

- Regular Physical Activity: Engage in regular physical activity as advised by your healthcare provider. Aim for at least 150 minutes of moderate-intensity aerobic exercise per week, or as recommended for your specific health condition. Consult with your healthcare team before starting any exercise program.

- Stress Management: Practice stress management techniques such as deep breathing exercises, meditation, yoga, or engaging in activities you find relaxing. Chronic stress can contribute to cardiovascular problems, so finding healthy ways to cope with stress is important.

3. Regular Medical Monitoring:

- Attend regular check-ups and follow-up appointments with your healthcare provider. They can monitor your blood pressure, cholesterol levels, kidney function, and overall cardiovascular health. They may also adjust medications or treatment plans as necessary.

- Medication Adherence: Take your prescribed medications as directed and follow the recommended dosage schedule. Do not discontinue or alter medications without consulting your healthcare provider.

Remember, individual approaches may vary depending on your specific health condition and recommendations from your healthcare provider. It's important to work closely with your healthcare team to develop a personalized plan for managing hypertension and promoting cardiovascular health in the context of CKD.

# 6.

# Creating a Supportive Environment

Creating a supportive environment is crucial for individuals living with Chronic Kidney Disease (CKD) to promote overall well-being and enhance their quality of life. Here are some considerations for fostering a supportive environment:

1. Education and Awareness: Educate family members, friends, and close contacts about CKD, its impact on daily life, and the importance of support. Help them understand the challenges and adjustments you may need to make, such as dietary restrictions,

medication schedules, and the need for regular medical appointments.

2. Communication: Maintain open and honest communication with your loved ones about your needs, concerns, and any changes in your health. Express how they can support you effectively, whether it's through emotional support, assistance with daily tasks, or accompanying you to medical appointments.

3. Emotional Support: Seek emotional support from family, friends, or support groups. They can provide a listening ear, empathy, and encouragement during difficult times. Joining online or in-person support groups specific to CKD can connect you with others who understand your journey and can offer valuable insights and support.

4. Practical Support: Allow your support system to assist you with practical tasks, such as grocery shopping, meal preparation, or transportation to medical appointments. Accepting help can alleviate some of the burdens and allow you to focus on self-care and managing your health.

5. Lifestyle Modifications Together: Involve your loved ones in your lifestyle modifications, such as dietary changes or incorporating exercise into your routine. Encourage them to adopt healthier habits alongside you, promoting a supportive and healthier environment for everyone.

6. Encourage Active Participation: Invite your family or close friends to learn more about CKD and be involved in your care. Encourage them to attend medical appointments, ask questions, and gain a better understanding of your treatment plan. This involvement can

foster a sense of shared responsibility and
support.

7. Patience and Understanding: Recognize that
adjustments and lifestyle changes can be
challenging for both you and your loved ones.
Practice patience and understanding as you
navigate this journey together. Provide
opportunities for open dialogue and address
any concerns or misconceptions that may
arise.

8. Celebrate Achievements: Acknowledge and
celebrate milestones and achievements in your
CKD management, such as improved lab
results or successfully adhering to dietary
recommendations. Share these victories with
your support system, as their encouragement
can motivate and uplift you.

9. Professional Support: Engage with healthcare professionals, including nephrologists, dietitians, and social workers, who can provide guidance and resources for creating a supportive environment. They can offer insights into caregiver support programs, community resources, and other services that may be beneficial to you and your loved ones.

Remember that building a supportive environment is an ongoing process that requires open communication, empathy, and collaboration. By involving your loved ones and fostering a sense of togetherness, you can create an environment that promotes your well-being and helps you manage the challenges of living with CKD more effectively.

# 7.

# Herbal and Dietary Supplements for Kidney Health

When it comes to herbal and dietary supplements for kidney health, it is essential to exercise caution and consult with your healthcare provider or a registered dietitian who specializes in kidney disease. While some supplements may have potential benefits, others can be harmful or interact with medications. Here are a few supplements that have been studied in relation to kidney health:

1. Omega-3 Fatty Acids: Found in fish oil and flaxseed oil, omega-3 fatty acids have anti-inflammatory properties and may have potential benefits for kidney health. However, the evidence is limited, and dosage recommendations may vary. Consult your

healthcare provider before starting any omega-3 fatty acid supplement.

2. Coenzyme Q10 (CoQ10): CoQ10 is an antioxidant that is naturally produced by the body and helps in energy production within cells. Some studies suggest that CoQ10 may have a protective effect on the kidneys. However, more research is needed to establish its efficacy and safety in kidney disease. Consult with your healthcare provider before taking CoQ10 supplements.

3. Probiotics: Probiotics are beneficial bacteria that promote a healthy gut microbiome. Some studies have shown that certain probiotics may have a positive impact on kidney function and reduce the risk of complications. However, specific strains and dosages have not been established, and more research is needed in this area.

4. Vitamin D: Vitamin D plays a crucial role in maintaining bone health and supporting the immune system. People with kidney disease often have low levels of vitamin D. Your healthcare provider may recommend vitamin D supplements to help maintain adequate levels. However, supplementation should be done under medical supervision, as excessive vitamin D intake can be harmful.

It is important to note that the use of herbal supplements and dietary supplements should be approached with caution, especially in the context of kidney disease. Many herbal supplements and over-the-counter products are not regulated by the FDA, and their safety and effectiveness may not be well-established.

Always talk to your healthcare provider before starting any new supplement, as they can evaluate your specific health condition, medications, and potential interactions or contraindications. They can provide personalized recommendations based on your individual needs and guide you towards evidence-based approaches for kidney health.

# 7.2

# Acupuncture and Traditional Chinese Medicine

Acupuncture and Traditional Chinese Medicine (TCM) are alternative therapies that have been used for centuries to promote health and treat various conditions, including kidney disease. Here is an overview of acupuncture and TCM in relation to kidney health:

1. Acupuncture: Acupuncture involves the insertion of thin needles into specific points on the body to stimulate energy flow and restore balance. Some potential benefits of acupuncture for kidney health include:

- Pain Management: Acupuncture may help alleviate pain associated with conditions such as chronic kidney disease, kidney stones, or urinary tract infections. It can provide relief from back pain, joint pain, and muscle tension.

- Stress Reduction: Acupuncture is believed to promote relaxation and reduce stress, which can be beneficial for individuals with kidney disease. Chronic stress can impact overall health and contribute to the progression of kidney disease.

- Symptom Management: Acupuncture may help manage symptoms related to kidney disease, such as fatigue, nausea, and insomnia.

It's important to note that while some studies suggest potential benefits, the scientific evidence supporting the use of acupuncture for kidney health is limited. It is recommended to consult with a qualified acupuncturist who has experience working with individuals with kidney disease and to discuss the potential risks and benefits before pursuing acupuncture as a treatment option.

2. Traditional Chinese Medicine (TCM): TCM is a comprehensive medical system that includes various modalities such as herbal medicine, acupuncture, dietary therapy, and lifestyle recommendations. In TCM, the emphasis restoring balance and harmony within the body to promote overall health. Some aspects of TCM that may be relevant to kidney health include:

   - Herbal Medicine: Traditional Chinese herbal formulas may be prescribed to support kidney function, address specific symptoms, or promote overall well-being. It is important to consult with a qualified herbalist or TCM practitioner who has experience working with kidney disease and to inform your healthcare provider about any herbal supplements you are taking, as they may interact with medications.

   - Dietary Therapy: TCM emphasizes the importance of a balanced diet tailored to an individual's specific needs. Dietary recommendations in TCM may focus on nourishing the kidneys, promoting fluid balance, and supporting overall health. Working with a registered dietitian who is knowledgeable about TCM principles can help ensure a proper integration of dietary therapy with medical recommendations for kidney disease.

   TCM is a complex system that requires expertise and individualized treatment. It is essential to consult with qualified practitioners who are experienced in working with kidney disease and to integrate TCM practices into a comprehensive treatment plan under the guidance of your healthcare provider.

It's important to note that while acupuncture and TCM may have potential benefits for some individuals, they should not replace conventional medical treatments for kidney disease. Always consult with your healthcare provider before starting any alternative therapies to ensure they are safe and appropriate for your specific condition.

# 7.3

# Yoga, Meditation, and Mindfulness Practices

Yoga, meditation, and mindfulness practices are complementary approaches that can provide numerous benefits for individuals with Chronic Kidney Disease (CKD). Here's an overview of these practices and their potential advantages:

1. Yoga: Yoga is a mind-body practice that combines physical postures, breathing exercises, and meditation. It offers several benefits for individuals with CKD, including:

- Physical Well-being: Yoga poses (asanas) can help improve flexibility, strength, and posture. It may also enhance circulation and reduce muscle tension.

- Stress Reduction: The combination of breath control and mindful movement in yoga can help reduce stress and promote relaxation. Chronic stress can negatively impact kidney health, and managing stress is essential for overall well-being.

- Blood Pressure Control: Some studies suggest that practicing yoga regularly may help lower blood pressure, which is important for individuals with hypertension, a common complication of CKD.

  - Improved Sleep: Yoga practices, especially relaxation techniques and gentle stretching before bedtime, can promote better sleep quality, which is important for overall health and well-being.

2. Meditation: Meditation involves focusing the mind and cultivating a state of deep awareness and relaxation. It can be beneficial for individuals with CKD in the following ways:

  - Stress Reduction: Meditation helps calm the mind and reduce stress, fostering a sense of peace and relaxation. Chronic stress can negatively impact kidney function, so managing stress is crucial.

  - Emotional Well-being: Meditation practices can enhance emotional well-being, reduce anxiety and depression symptoms, and promote a positive outlook on life. This can be particularly helpful for individuals dealing with the challenges of living with a chronic illness.

- Blood Pressure Control: Some studies suggest that regular meditation practice may help lower blood pressure levels, which is beneficial for individuals with hypertension.

3. Mindfulness Practices: Mindfulness involves paying attention to the present moment, without judgment or attachment. It can be practiced during daily activities and incorporated into various aspects of life. Benefits of mindfulness for individuals with CKD include:

- Stress Reduction: Mindfulness practices cultivate an attitude of acceptance and non-reactivity to stressors, helping individuals manage stress more effectively.

- Improved Emotional Well-being:
Mindfulness can enhance emotional resilience,
reduce anxiety and depression symptoms, and
promote a greater sense of overall well-being.

- Better Self-Care: Being mindful can help
individuals make healthier choices and engage
in self-care activities that support kidney
health, such as adhering to medication
schedules, following dietary restrictions, and
maintaining a regular exercise routine.

These practices can be integrated into your
daily routine, but it's important to consult with
your healthcare provider before starting any
new physical or mindfulness practices,
especially if you have specific health concerns
or limitations. They can provide guidance and
ensure that these practices are safe and
appropriate for your individual needs.

It's worth noting that yoga, meditation, and mindfulness practices should not replace medical treatments or advice. They can be used as complementary approaches to enhance overall well-being and support the management of CKD.

# 8.

# Fostering Resilience and Hope

Fostering resilience and maintaining a sense of hope is crucial for individuals living with Chronic Kidney Disease (CKD). Here are some strategies to help cultivate resilience and foster hope:

1. Educate Yourself: Gain knowledge about CKD, its treatment options, and how to manage the condition effectively. Understanding your condition can help you feel more empowered and in control of your health. Stay informed about the latest

advancements in kidney health and treatment options.

2. Set Realistic Goals: Set realistic short-term and long-term goals that are attainable and align with your health condition. These goals can be related to your treatment plan, lifestyle changes, or personal achievements. Celebrate your progress and small victories along the way.

3. Develop a Supportive Network: Surround yourself with a supportive network of family, friends, and healthcare professionals who understand your journey and provide encouragement. Joining support groups or online communities specific to CKD can also connect you with individuals who can relate to your experiences and provide support and hope.

4. Practice Self-Care: Prioritize self-care activities that contribute to your overall well-being. Engage in activities you enjoy, such as hobbies, exercise, or spending time with loved ones. Take breaks when needed, practice relaxation techniques, and ensure you are getting adequate rest and sleep.

5. Practice Mindfulness and Gratitude: Cultivate mindfulness by staying present in the moment and practicing gratitude for the things you have. Focus on the positive aspects of your life, express gratitude for small victories, and appreciate the support and care you receive.

6. Maintain a Healthy Lifestyle: Adhere to your treatment plan, including medications, dietary recommendations, and exercise routines. A healthy lifestyle can contribute to your overall well-being and potentially slow down the progression of CKD. Consult with your

healthcare provider or a registered dietitian for personalized guidance.

7. Seek Emotional Support: If you find yourself struggling emotionally, consider seeking professional help. A mental health professional can provide guidance, coping strategies, and support to help you navigate the emotional challenges of living with CKD.

8. Stay Hopeful and Optimistic: Cultivate a positive mindset and remain hopeful about your future. Focus on the opportunities that lie ahead, the advancements in medical research, and the potential for improved treatments. Stay engaged in activities that bring you joy and provide a sense of purpose.

9. Practice Resilience: Embrace resilience by recognizing that setbacks and challenges are part of the journey. Learn from them, adapt,

and bounce back stronger. Develop coping mechanisms and problem-solving skills to navigate obstacles along the way.

Remember that resilience and hope are ongoing practices that require continuous effort and self-care. Embrace the support available to you, stay informed, and focus on maintaining a positive outlook. Your ability to foster resilience and maintain hope can make a significant difference in managing CKD and living a fulfilling life.

# 8.1

# Celebrating Small Victories and Milestones

Celebrating small victories and milestones is an important aspect of living with Chronic Kidney Disease (CKD) and can contribute to a positive mindset and overall well-being. Here are some ways to celebrate and acknowledge your achievements:

1. Set Meaningful Goals: Set specific, realistic goals that are meaningful to you. These goals can be related to your health, treatment plan, lifestyle changes, or personal achievements. Break them down into smaller, achievable steps. Celebrate each milestone you reach along the way.

2. Reflect on Progress: Take time to reflect on your progress regularly. Acknowledge how far you've come and the positive changes you've made. It can be helpful to keep a journal or log to track your accomplishments and milestones, both big and small.

3. Reward Yourself: Treat yourself to small rewards as you achieve your goals. It could be something simple like enjoying a favorite meal, indulging in a hobby or activity you love, or taking time for self-care, such as a relaxing bath or a massage. These rewards can serve as reminders of your achievements and provide motivation to continue moving forward.

4. Share with Loved Ones: Share your victories and milestones with your loved ones. Celebrate with your family and friends, and allow them to share in your joy and success. Their support and encouragement can boost your morale and strengthen your bond with them.

5. Practice Gratitude: Express gratitude for the progress you've made and the milestones you've achieved. Take a moment each day to

reflect on the positive aspects of your life and the blessings you have. Cultivating a sense of gratitude can shift your focus towards the positive and enhance your overall well-being.

6. Celebrate Non-Health Related Achievements: It's important to celebrate achievements beyond your health. Recognize and celebrate accomplishments in other areas of your life, such as work, hobbies, relationships, or personal growth. This broadens your perspective and helps you maintain a balanced and fulfilling life.

7. Join Supportive Communities: Connect with support groups or online communities specifically for individuals with CKD. Share your milestones and celebrate with others who can relate to your experiences. These communities provide a space for mutual support, encouragement, and celebration.

8. Practice Self-Reflection: Take time to reflect on your journey and the challenges you've overcome. Recognize your strength and resilience. Use these reflections as a reminder of your ability to overcome obstacles and to inspire yourself to keep pushing forward.

Remember, celebrating small victories and milestones is not about the size of the achievement but about recognizing and appreciating your progress. It's an opportunity to acknowledge your efforts, boost your motivation, and maintain a positive outlook on your journey with CKD.

# 9.

# Travel and Lifestyle Considerations, Tips for Safe Travel with CKD

Traveling with Chronic Kidney Disease (CKD) requires some additional planning and considerations to ensure your safety and well-being. Here are some tips to help you have a safe and enjoyable travel experience:

1. Consult with Your Healthcare Team: Before planning your trip, consult with your healthcare team, including your nephrologist or healthcare provider. They can assess your current health status, provide guidance specific to your condition, and advise you on any necessary precautions or adjustments.

2. Plan Ahead: Research your destination and
ensure that it can accommodate your specific
needs. Look for healthcare facilities in the area
and have a plan in case of emergencies.
Consider the availability of dialysis centers or
medical professionals who specialize in kidney
care, if needed.

3. Medication and Supplies: Make sure you
have an ample supply of your medications,
including any prescriptions, and pack them in
your carry-on bag. Carry a list of your
medications, their dosages, and any specific
instructions from your healthcare provider.
Consider bringing extra supplies such as
bandages, wound care items, and
disinfectants.

4. Stay Hydrated: Adequate hydration is crucial
for individuals with CKD. Carry a refillable

water bottle and drink plenty of water throughout your journey. Be mindful of the water quality at your destination and consider using bottled or filtered water for drinking and brushing your teeth.

5. Stick to Your Dietary Restrictions: If you follow a specific dietary plan, try to adhere to it as much as possible while traveling. Pack snacks or meals that align with your dietary needs, especially during long flights or train rides. Research local food options that are kidney-friendly and communicate any dietary restrictions or allergies to restaurant staff.

6. Maintain a Healthy Lifestyle: Despite being on vacation, continue to prioritize a healthy lifestyle. Follow your exercise routine, practice stress-reducing techniques, and get enough restful sleep. Engaging in physical activity and managing stress can help maintain your overall well-being while traveling.

7. Protect Yourself: Take precautions to protect your health during your journey. Wash your hands frequently, use hand sanitizers when necessary, and avoid close contact with individuals who may be sick. Follow local guidelines and recommendations regarding face coverings and social distancing.

8. Travel Insurance: Consider obtaining travel insurance that covers medical emergencies and expenses related to your CKD. Review the policy carefully to ensure it meets your specific needs and provides adequate coverage for your condition.

9. Pace Yourself: Traveling can be physically demanding, so pace yourself and listen to your body. Take breaks when needed and avoid overexertion. Allow time for rest and

relaxation to prevent fatigue and ensure you can enjoy your trip fully.

10. Enjoy the Experience: Remember to have fun and enjoy your travel experience. Take time to immerse yourself in the local culture, connect with the people you meet, and create lasting memories. Traveling can be a rewarding and enriching experience, and with proper planning, you can make it an enjoyable one while managing your CKD.

Always consult with your healthcare provider before making any travel plans to ensure that it is safe for you to travel based on your individual health condition and needs. They can provide personalized guidance and recommendations specific to your situation.

# 9.1

# Balancing Work and Lifestyle Demands

Balancing work and lifestyle demands is crucial for individuals living with Chronic Kidney Disease (CKD) to maintain their overall well-being. Here are some strategies to help you find balance:

1. Communicate with Your Employer: Openly communicate with your employer about your health condition and any specific needs or accommodations you may require. Discuss flexible work arrangements, such as modified work hours or remote work options, if feasible. Inform them about any medical appointments or treatments that may require time off or adjustments to your schedule.

2. Prioritize Self-Care: Make self-care a priority in your daily routine. Set aside time for activities that promote your physical and emotional well-being, such as exercise, relaxation techniques, hobbies, and spending time with loved ones. Taking care of yourself will enhance your ability to manage work demands and cope with the challenges of CKD.

3. Manage Stress: Chronic illness and work-related stress can take a toll on your well-being. Implement stress management techniques, such as deep breathing exercises, meditation, or mindfulness practices. Identify stress triggers in your work environment and develop strategies to cope with them effectively.

4. Set Realistic Work Expectations: Be realistic about what you can accomplish within your

work responsibilities. Prioritize tasks and focus on the most critical ones. Delegate when appropriate and communicate with your colleagues and supervisors about workload adjustments, if needed.

5. Take Regular Breaks: Incorporate regular breaks into your workday to recharge and avoid burnout. Use these breaks to stretch, relax, or engage in activities that help you decompress. Stepping away from work periodically can improve productivity and overall well-being.

6. Advocate for Yourself: Be your own advocate in the workplace. Communicate your needs and limitations to your colleagues and supervisors. Educate them about CKD and how it may impact your work. Request reasonable accommodations, if necessary, to ensure you can perform your job duties effectively.

7. Time Management: Effectively manage your time to balance work and personal responsibilities. Prioritize tasks and create a schedule that allows for breaks, medical appointments, and self-care activities. Avoid overcommitting and learn to say no when necessary to avoid overwhelming yourself.

8. Seek Support: Reach out for support from your healthcare team, family, friends, or support groups. They can provide emotional support, understanding, and practical advice on managing work and lifestyle demands. Connecting with others who may be facing similar challenges can be reassuring and empowering.

9. Know Your Rights: Familiarize yourself with the employment laws and policies that protect individuals with chronic illnesses. Understand

your rights related to accommodations, leave of absence, and other workplace protections. Consult with human resources or seek legal advice if you encounter any issues or challenges in the workplace.

Remember, finding balance between work and lifestyle demands is an ongoing process. It may require adjustments, communication, and self-care strategies tailored to your specific situation. Prioritize your health and well-being, and seek the necessary support to help you navigate the challenges and maintain a fulfilling work-life balance with CKD.

# 10.

# Preventing CKD Progression and Future

Preventing the progression of Chronic Kidney Disease (CKD) and maintaining a positive future outlook is crucial for managing the condition effectively. Here are some key strategies to consider:

1. Medical Management: Work closely with your healthcare team to manage your CKD. This includes regular check-ups, monitoring kidney function, and adjusting treatment plans as needed. Adhere to medication regimens, follow dietary guidelines, and make necessary lifestyle changes to control underlying conditions like diabetes and hypertension.

2. Blood Pressure Control: High blood pressure can accelerate kidney damage. Monitor your blood pressure regularly and work with your healthcare provider to maintain it within a healthy range. This may involve lifestyle modifications, such as reducing sodium intake, exercising regularly, and taking prescribed medications.

3. Blood Sugar Control: If you have diabetes, it's crucial to keep your blood sugar levels under control. Consistently monitor your blood glucose levels, follow a diabetes management plan, and take any prescribed medications. Keeping your blood sugar stable can help slow the progression of CKD.

4. Healthy Lifestyle Habits: Adopting healthy lifestyle habits can positively impact your kidney health. Maintain a balanced diet that is

low in sodium, saturated fats, and processed foods. Stay physically active by engaging in regular exercise, as recommended by your healthcare provider. Avoid smoking and limit alcohol consumption.

5. Regular Exercise: Engaging in regular physical activity can have numerous benefits for your overall health, including kidney health. Talk to your healthcare provider about suitable exercise options for your condition. Aim for a combination of cardiovascular exercises, strength training, and flexibility exercises.

6. Stay Hydrated: Adequate hydration is essential for kidney health. Drink enough water throughout the day to stay hydrated, unless your healthcare provider has recommended specific fluid restrictions. Remember to balance your fluid intake

according to your kidney function and any recommendations from your healthcare team.

7. Regular Monitoring and Screening: Stay proactive in monitoring your kidney function by regularly undergoing urine and blood tests. These tests help your healthcare provider assess your kidney health and detect any changes or abnormalities early on. Early detection and intervention can help slow the progression of CKD.

8. Mental and Emotional Health: Take care of your mental and emotional well-being. Living with CKD can be challenging, so prioritize activities that promote stress reduction, relaxation, and emotional well-being. Consider joining support groups, seeking counseling, or practicing mindfulness and stress-management techniques.

9. Educate Yourself and Stay Informed: Continually educate yourself about CKD, its management, and any advancements in treatment options. Stay informed about lifestyle changes, dietary recommendations, and new developments in kidney health research. This knowledge empowers you to make informed decisions and take an active role in your care.

Remember that every individual's journey with CKD is unique, and the progression of the disease can vary. With proper management, lifestyle modifications, and ongoing support from your healthcare team, you can take steps to slow the progression of CKD and maintain a positive future outlook.

# 10. 1

# Early intervention and preventive measures

Early intervention and preventive measures play a crucial role in managing and potentially slowing the progression of Chronic Kidney Disease (CKD). Here are some key strategies for early intervention and prevention:

1. Regular Health Check-ups: Schedule regular check-ups with your healthcare provider to monitor your kidney function and overall health. Routine screenings, such as blood pressure measurements and urine tests, can help identify early signs of kidney problems and allow for timely intervention.

2. Manage Underlying Conditions: Properly manage underlying health conditions that can contribute to the development or progression of CKD, such as diabetes and hypertension. Follow your healthcare provider's recommendations for medications, lifestyle modifications, and regular monitoring to keep these conditions under control.

3. Healthy Lifestyle Habits: Adopt a healthy lifestyle to reduce the risk of kidney disease. Maintain a balanced diet that is low in sodium, saturated fats, and processed foods. Eat plenty of fruits, vegetables, whole grains, and lean proteins. Engage in regular physical activity, maintain a healthy weight, avoid smoking, and limit alcohol consumption.

4. Blood Pressure Control: High blood pressure (hypertension) is a leading cause of kidney disease. Monitor your blood pressure regularly and work with your healthcare provider to

keep it within a healthy range. Lifestyle changes, such as reducing sodium intake, regular exercise, and prescribed medications, may be necessary to achieve and maintain optimal blood pressure levels.

5. Blood Sugar Control: If you have diabetes, it's essential to manage your blood sugar levels effectively. Monitor your blood glucose levels regularly, follow a diabetes management plan, and take prescribed medications as directed. Maintaining stable blood sugar levels can help prevent or slow the progression of kidney disease.

6. Avoid Nephrotoxic Substances: Be cautious about substances that can be harmful to the kidneys. Non-prescription pain medications, such as nonsteroidal anti-inflammatory drugs (NSAIDs), and certain herbal supplements can have adverse effects on kidney function.

Always consult with your healthcare provider before taking any medications or supplements.

7. Stay Hydrated: Proper hydration is important for kidney health. Drink an adequate amount of water throughout the day, unless you have specific fluid restrictions recommended by your healthcare provider. Adequate hydration helps maintain optimal kidney function and prevents the formation of kidney stones.

8. Avoid Self-Medication: Avoid self-medicating or taking over-the-counter medications without consulting your healthcare provider. Some medications, including certain painkillers and herbal remedies, can be harmful to the kidneys, especially when taken inappropriately or in excessive amounts.

9. Educate Yourself: Educate yourself about CKD, its risk factors, and preventive measures. Stay informed about the importance of regular screenings, early intervention, and lifestyle modifications. Understand the signs and symptoms of kidney disease to seek medical attention promptly if needed.

10. Genetic Testing: In certain cases, genetic testing may be recommended, especially for individuals with a family history of kidney disease. Genetic testing can help identify any inherited conditions that may increase the risk of kidney problems and allow for early intervention and management.

Remember, early intervention and preventive measures are crucial in managing CKD. By proactively addressing risk factors, adopting a healthy lifestyle, and seeking appropriate medical care, you can potentially slow the progression of kidney disease and improve your long-term kidney health. Regular communication with your healthcare provider and adherence to their recommendations are key to effective early intervention and prevention.

# 11

# Embracing the Journey to Wellness with CKD

Embracing the journey to wellness with Chronic Kidney Disease (CKD) is an ongoing process that involves making positive changes, adopting a proactive mindset, and finding balance in various aspects of life. Here are some key points to consider in embracing the journey to wellness with CKD:

1. Acceptance and Education: Acknowledge and accept your diagnosis of CKD. Take the time to educate yourself about the condition, its causes, and its management strategies. Understanding the disease empowers you to make informed decisions and actively participate in your treatment plan.

2. Self-Care and Lifestyle Modifications: Prioritize self-care by making healthy lifestyle modifications. Follow a kidney-friendly diet, manage fluid intake, engage in regular physical activity as recommended by your healthcare provider, and get enough rest and sleep. These lifestyle changes can help slow the progression of CKD and improve overall well-being.

3. Building a Support Network: Surround yourself with a supportive network of family, friends, and healthcare professionals who understand and empathize with your journey. Join support groups, both online and offline, to

connect with others facing similar challenges. Sharing experiences, exchanging advice, and receiving encouragement can make a significant difference in your well-being.

4. Communication with Healthcare Providers: Establish open and honest communication with your healthcare providers. Share any concerns, symptoms, or challenges you may be experiencing. Collaborate with them to create a personalized treatment plan that addresses your specific needs and goals.

5. Emotional and Mental Health: Prioritize your emotional and mental well-being. Living with CKD can bring about various emotions, such as stress, anxiety, and depression. Seek support from mental health professionals, participate in counseling or therapy, and practice stress management techniques such as meditation, mindfulness, and relaxation exercises.

6. Adherence to Treatment Plan: Follow your healthcare provider's instructions regarding medications, dietary restrictions, and lifestyle recommendations. Consistent adherence to your treatment plan is vital for managing CKD effectively and optimizing kidney health.

7. Regular Monitoring and Check-ups: Attend regular check-ups and monitoring appointments with your healthcare provider. These visits allow for the evaluation of your kidney function, adjustments to treatment plans if necessary, and the early detection of any complications or changes in your condition.

8. Celebrate Progress and Small Victories: Acknowledge and celebrate your progress and small victories along the journey. Whether it's achieving personal health goals, maintaining

stable kidney function, or successfully implementing positive lifestyle changes, recognize and reward yourself for your efforts and achievements.

9. Finding Meaning and Purpose: Explore ways to find meaning and purpose in your life despite the challenges posed by CKD. Engage in activities that bring joy and fulfillment, pursue hobbies or interests, and set realistic goals that align with your current capabilities and priorities.

Remember, embracing the journey to wellness with CKD is a personal and individual process. It requires patience, resilience, and a commitment to self-care. By taking an active role in your own health, seeking support, and maintaining a positive mindset, you can navigate the challenges of CKD while striving for overall well-being and a fulfilling life.

# 11.1

# Empowering Yourself for a Fulfilling Life

Empowering yourself for a fulfilling life while living with Chronic Kidney Disease (CKD) involves taking control of your health, making informed decisions, and embracing a proactive mindset. Here are some key strategies to empower yourself for a fulfilling life with CKD:

1. Education and Knowledge: Educate yourself about CKD, its causes, symptoms, and available treatment options. Stay informed about the latest research and advancements in kidney health. Understanding your condition empowers you to actively participate in your care and make informed decisions.

2. Open Communication with Healthcare Providers: Develop a strong and open relationship with your healthcare team. Communicate your concerns, ask questions, and seek clarification about your treatment plan. Be an active participant in discussions about your health and collaborate with your healthcare providers to make decisions that align with your goals.

3. Self-Advocacy: Advocate for yourself and your needs. Be proactive in managing your health by scheduling regular check-ups, monitoring your symptoms, and reporting any changes or concerns to your healthcare providers. Speak up about your preferences and priorities in your treatment plan.

4. Building a Support System: Surround yourself with a supportive network of family, friends, and fellow CKD patients. Join support groups, both online and offline, where you can

share experiences, exchange advice, and receive emotional support. Connecting with others who understand your journey can be empowering and provide a sense of community.

5. Self-Care and Lifestyle Management: Prioritize self-care and implement healthy lifestyle habits. Follow a kidney-friendly diet, engage in regular physical activity, get enough rest and sleep, manage stress, and practice relaxation techniques. Taking care of your physical and mental well-being enhances your quality of life and empowers you to better manage your condition.

6. Setting Realistic Goals: Set realistic goals that align with your capabilities and priorities. Break down larger goals into smaller, achievable steps. Celebrate each milestone and progress along the way. Setting and achieving goals boosts your confidence,

motivation, and overall sense of empowerment.

7. Seeking Emotional Support: Take care of your emotional well-being. Living with CKD can bring about various emotions. Seek support from mental health professionals, participate in therapy or counseling, and practice stress management techniques. Emotional support can help you cope with challenges, improve your mental health, and enhance your overall well-being.

8. Continuing Education and Self-Improvement: Stay engaged in lifelong learning and personal development. Attend educational workshops or webinars related to CKD, join patient education programs, and stay up to date with relevant research and advancements. Continuously expanding your knowledge empowers you to make informed decisions and actively manage your health.

9. Finding Meaning and Purpose: Seek meaning and purpose in your life beyond CKD. Engage in activities, hobbies, or interests that bring you joy, fulfillment, and a sense of purpose. Cultivate meaningful relationships, pursue personal goals, and contribute to causes or communities that are important to you. Focusing on what brings you happiness and fulfillment can empower you to live a fulfilling life despite the challenges of CKD.

Remember, empowerment is an ongoing process, and it may look different for each individual. By taking charge of your health, seeking support, staying informed, and embracing a proactive mindset, you can empower yourself to lead a fulfilling life with CKD. Embrace your personal strengths, nurture your well-being, and strive for a life that is meaningful and satisfying to you is on